Living
MIGRAINE
FREE!

My breakthrough discovery

Allan McMullen

ISBN-13: 978-1461034094
ISBN-10: 1461034094

Illustrations: Tom Fagan
Copyediting and book design: Kenneth Guentert, The Publishing Pro, LLC, Colorado Springs, Colorado

Contents

Preface

Our knowledge comes from a variety of sources: what our parents taught us, what we learned in school, what we've read, seen or believe to be true, and, of course, personal experiences. It's hard to say if one source is more valid than another, but certainly, we draw from all of them as we go through life.

We are constantly seeking answers from this knowledge base to resolve things and move forward. Within this process of acquiring and recombining information, new understanding is formed. Breakthroughs happen, we just need to embrace that moment and assimilate its meaning.

Knowledge from all of the above sources is used in this book. I am not a doctor, I'm the case study who discovered a way through the turmoil and back out into the sunshine. Though our bodies operate basically the same way, we all have different tolerances. If this book helps you, then celebrate, if it doesn't, keep searching. This is a guidebook to better health, and I hope there is a breakthrough waiting somewhere in there, for you.—A.M.

As I was working on this book, I noticed that the more I wrote "migraine headache" the more I felt its presence. As a result, I thought it would be wise to avoid the power of suggestion on myself and my readers, and so began referring to a migraine headache as "an MH."

The techniques and recommendations in this book are intended to enhance the body's natural ability to heal itself and to supplement other forms of medical treatment. Seek professional medical advice if pain persists.

My Story

Like many other people in the world, I have suffered from migraine headaches since childhood and know what it is like to live with such a strange and debilitating ailment. The staggering number of migraine cases and the extent of the pain endured by so many has prompted me to write about what I've learned in my search for a cure. I too would still be living a life distorted by migraines if it were not for the amazing discovery that has freed me from their grip.

The cause and cure for my migraine headaches were always somewhat of a mystery to me. The various doctors I saw offered different explanations, but the drugs they prescribed had adverse side affects and didn't provide any lasting relief. Avoiding certain foods didn't help either. Nothing seemed to work on these headaches, and I was left only with the hope that one day I would outgrow them. Unfortunately, that day never came.

Time soon found me well into my thirties with no available cure. Motivated by desperation, I resolved to find one on my own. Through self-analysis and personal research, I slowly identified certain behavioral patterns and triggers for my headaches. A better understanding of my reactions to stress helped me to adapt and to reduce the frequency of migraines, but I still didn't have a cure. The answer eluded me until one day I discovered it quite by accident. Finally, I had a way to either neutralize a migraine at its onset or shut it down once it started. The cure was not a drug but a simple and natural breathing exercise.

Here are the tried and true facts that have successfully helped me and many other migraine sufferers regain a healthy existence. Today, these headaches are no longer of such monster proportions in my life. With my discovery, migraines no longer control me, I control them. It is my sincere wish that you too will be able to free yourself from migraine headaches after reading this book.

Before going any further, I want to make sure that I avoid the power of suggestion on readers who suffer from migraines and so will refer to a migraine headache from this point forward simply as an MH.

What Is an MH?

WHAT IS AN MH? Most medical descriptions of an MH indicate that it is the result of abnormal expansion and contraction of blood vessels in and around the brain. The expansion or dilation of the vessels and the associated nerve pain make an MH different from a tension headache. The resulting symptoms vary, depending on the individual and the intensity of the MH. I experience a super-sensitivity to light and sound, partial hearing loss in one ear, throbbing head pain, dizziness, and distorted vision and balance. Certainly, what makes an MH so brutal is the potential severity or duration of the attack. I've had headaches that have put me in bed for days and others that have cycled in and out for weeks. I could never tell just how severe an MH was going to be until it ran its course.

What Causes an MH?

There are many theories for MH causes. Some of the more accepted explanations are that people susceptible to an MH perceive and define stress differently from other people; that MH sufferers have a more sensitive nervous system response; or that they have a heightened sense of concern, are easily alarmed, or are more emotionally reactive. There are certainly more explanations than these out there, but all of them can produce a downward spiral in the psyche of the individual. Often these responses trigger an associated "stress hormone" release within the body like the primal fight or flee reaction. For many people, these stress chemicals dissipate without lasting side effects, but for the MH sufferer they can trigger an MH. Menstrual cycles, diet, and fatigue also add to bio-chemical undulations. All of these contributors can lead vulnerable individuals down the road to an MH. It could be a tsunami style attack or a trickle build-up over time, but the process is the same. Negativity begins to over-whelm your peace of mind, which reduces your body's natural ability to repair and heal itself. This imbalance can propel you toward an MH, among other maladies. Your challenge as an MH sufferer is to avoid remaining sub-merged in the gloom of a negative state of mind, where sickness thrives, but to move back into the light of positive consciousness as soon as possible. Staying positive and optimistic blocks all of these nervous system response trig-gers and keeps you moving away from any kind of MH build-up.

The Onset Phase

Most people fail to recognize the subtle onset phase, which is the build-up to an MH. It is extremely important that you become attuned to the warning signals characteristic of the onset phase and take immediate action to ward off an attack. This phase can last for days, weeks, or longer. During this period, an MH can be more easily provoked. You may drift in and out of this phase without knowing of your increased exposure to an MH. This is a time when consuming certain foods like alcohol and sweets, or a confrontation with another person, may cause a full-blown MH.

The Warning Signals

The warning signals associated with the onset phase vary with each individual but tend to be subtle versions of sensations experienced during an MH. These uncomfortable sensations usually arrive in the same sequence, which can help you begin to recognize them. My initial symptom is a faint ringing or low pulsating hum in my ears. I perceive this sound most easily during the quiet moments of the day, such as first thing in the morning or at night. This symptom graduates into a dull swirling ache in the temples or the top half of my head and often leads to a sporadic swoon of imbalance or vertigo. Reduced hearing in one ear usually follows. Whatever *your* warning signals, don't ignore them. You can neutralize them with the following breathing exercise before they lead to an MH attack. Also keep in mind that after you think an MH has run its course, and you are returning to normal, you may instead find yourself back in the onset phase, once more experiencing your warning symptoms and an elevated vulnerability to another MH attack.

My Discovery

The Breathing Exercise

Years ago, when I was single and living by myself, I experienced a particularly vicious cycle of MH attacks that took place over several months. Desperate for relief, I retreated to nature and the peaceful mountains for some overnight camping. Though I was not having an MH at the time, I had the nagging symptoms that foreshadowed another MH. That evening, while sitting inside my tent blowing up an inflatable air mattress, I felt a soothing sensation in my head. Compared to all the throbbing head pain I had been feeling, this sensation caught my attention. The next day I awoke with a clear head. All the uncomfortable MH symptoms were gone. Was this the breakthrough I had been looking for?

I soon developed a breathing exercise based on my discovery of blowing up the air mattress and began using it to neutralize MHs with remarkable success. It proved to be the cure I was looking for, but it was so simple it took me a while to acknowledge the incredible results. This exercise is a natural alternative to medication, has no side affects, and can be done anywhere—at work, in the car, or in bed at night. Using this technique in concert with the other techniques in this book, I have been able to leave behind the painful world of the MH.

If you have ever tried to blow into a balloon or inflatable, you've probably experienced a feeling of back-pressure in your head. This sensation of back-pressure is the key that neutralizes an MH. No other kind of breathing achieves the same curative results.

Resistance Breathing

This exercise alone provides the resistance to your exhalation and the pacing to your breathing that normalizes the body.

Here is how you do the MH breathing exercise.

- Make a loose fist with one hand by bending the fingers down to the palm and then fold the thumb lightly over the top of the fingers.

- Press the end of your fist to your mouth with your thumb knuckle to one corner and the knuckle of your hand against the other corner of your mouth.

- Gently blow into that little hole as if you were blowing a long note on a trumpet. Adjust the opening in your fist so that you can exhale in this manner to a ten-count, with most of your breath expelled by the end of the count.

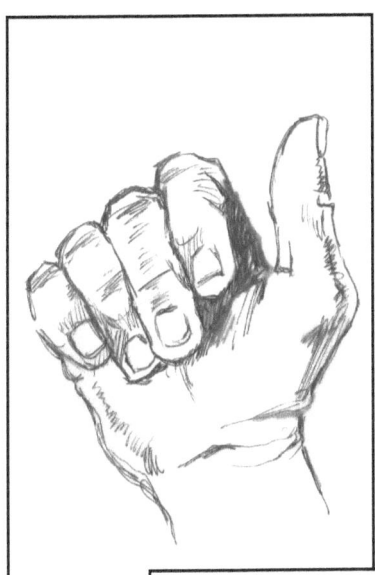

Make a loose fist with one hand by bending the fingers down to the palm and then fold the thumb lightly over the top of the fingers

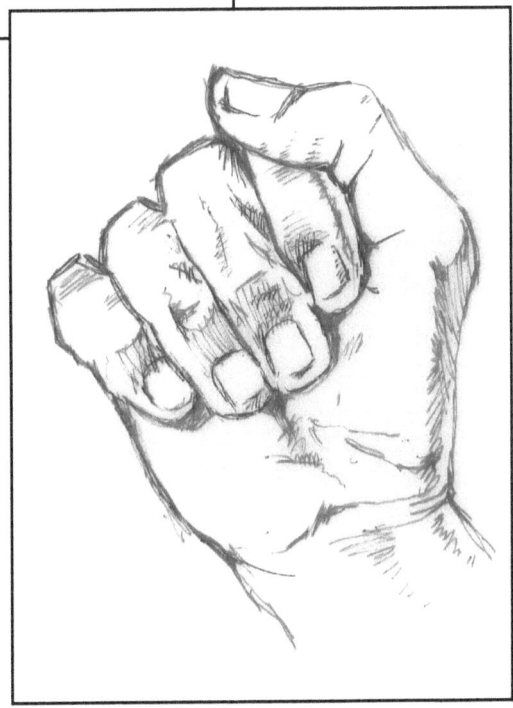

- Take another deep breath and repeat again.

The resistance to your exhale should be no greater than what is necessary to blow up a balloon. If your eyes feel like they are bulging out, then you are blowing too hard and the opening in your fist should be a little bigger. If you exhale all the air before the ten-count, then the opening in your fist needs to be smaller. Twenty exhale/inhale cycles in a row with gentle resistance is all that's necessary to achieve optimum results. You can repeat this resistance breathing exercise several times during the course of a day, and you definitely should repeat it if an MH is in progress.

I have found that bedtime is an excellent time to do this exercise because it neutralizes the accumulated stress of the day and allows sleep to come more easily. The idea is to always wake up clear with a stress-free head.

Considering all that you have been through, this breathing exercise may sound too simplistic to be effective. It is not a pill that immediately covers up pain. It is a natural way to specifically neutralize MH symptoms and attacks, and is an essential supplement to other types of MH medical treatments. If you give it a chance, it will work wonders for you as it has for me and many others. My life would have been much more difficult and painful over the years had it not been for my discovery of this miraculous resistance breathing exercise.

When Should You Do the Breathing Exercise?

If you are susceptible to MHs and experience a stressful event, you must anticipate an MH as a possible by-product and take preventive action, especially if onset symptoms appear. Do the breathing exercise as soon as possible or at least that night before going to sleep. I once recommended the exercise to a friend, who said she sometimes had several different MHs in a single day. Ten minutes after doing twenty repetitions of the resistance breathing exercise, she bounced into the room and proclaimed that her MH was gone. This was interesting to me because my MH experiences have always been at the more severe end of the spectrum, and I have never been able to end an MH in ten minutes. However, if I repeat the exercise several times in one day and get a good night's sleep, I usually wake up clear the next day. Your results may vary or be subtle when you first start using

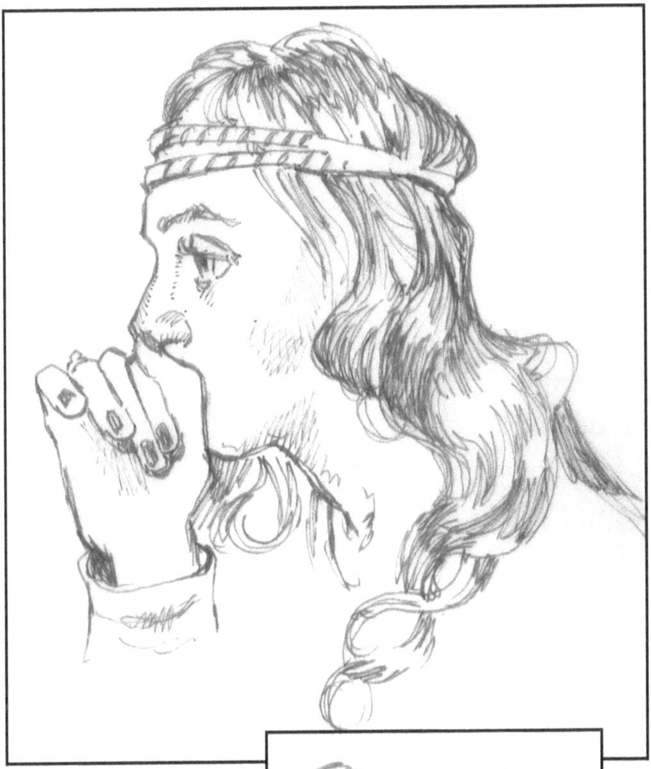

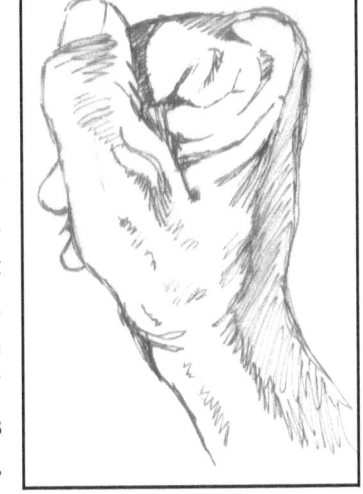

Your results may vary or be subtle when you first start using this exercise. Be patient. Try twenty repetitions every evening at bedtime for a week, and then develop an "as necessary" sequence that works best for you.

this exercise. Be patient. Try it every evening at bedtime for a week, and then develop an "as necessary" sequence that works best for you.

Once I became attuned to the onset phase of an MH, I realized that I usually have a lag time between a stressful occurrence and an MH attack, occasionally several days. Before I discovered this, I would sometimes be awakened in the middle of the night by the sheer force of a full-blown MH and wonder where it came from. Now I could neutralize the build up with the breathing exercise and avoid an MH attack altogether. This also helped me pinpoint the events and causes of my stress. As these correlations became more familiar to me, I realized I had the power to change my perception of what is worth stressing about and what is not.

Know Yourself

To learn when stress and tension are overwhelming you is to know when you are vulnerable to MH attacks. Some common examples of stress are:

■ Stress from an emotionally charged event made worse by internalizing negative feelings.

■ Stress accumulating over a period of time from a negative mental or emotional state. It may be so subtle you have ignored it, or it may be an obvious aggravation accompanied by fits of anger.

■ Stress from lack of human interaction often associated with idleness, loneliness, or fear about the future.

■ Night stress, caused by an inability to sleep deeply due to a mental or physical anxiety like worry or chronic pain. The body's ability to completely relax is compromised, resulting in restless sleep often accompanied by active or hostile dreams.

- Stress from the bad habit of repeated negative thinking.

The key is becoming responsive to "stress overloads" rather than letting them accumulate within you. What it all comes down to is taking the great mix of life that happens on a daily basis and staying mentally, physically, and emotionally in balance. This is a considerable challenge that requires continual awareness and practice. I have found that the following *centering techniques* are essential for maintaining this balance and staying free from the grip of an MH.

Coping with Change

Life is constantly changing and moving forward, which means that coping with life is primarily about coping with change. Sometimes the easiest route is to replace one kind of response with another, like replacing a negative view with a positive one. Is the glass half empty or half full? The answer determines whether you are on your way down or on your way up. It has been said that *90 percent of life is perception.* If you can reshape your thinking and focus on the positive instead of the negative, then you can deflect stress before it erodes your peace of mind. Negative thoughts and emotions come from negatively perceiving the reality of a situation. On the other hand, positive outlooks like insight, understanding, and compassion are more often free from distortion and allow you to think clearly and pursue an original and satisfying path. I believe that many negative interpretations of reality are nothing more than habits that I have acquired or absorbed from childhood until now. This realization started a behavioral evolution that enabled me to negate stress by turning off the negative voice inside my head in favor of the positive reassuring one. This positive inner voice is always available to you as well. It's the same one you'd use to console a discouraged child, support a friend in need, or cheer on your favorite team. Everyone has this powerful and supportive voice, but for some reason many people seldom use it on themselves. *Self-encouragement* through positive affirmation is one of the great secrets to success. It builds confidence and perseverance. Because life is dynamic, commitment to this sort of personal growth must continue for a lifetime. However, you can create fulfilling change in an instant, just as you would tune your radio to a more upbeat song.

Setting Goals

Without goals, you will have no forward progress. If you do nothing, you feel like nothing. Therefore, as the climbers say on Mount Everest, keep moving. Goals are what you are moving toward. They keep you focused. In this age of too many choices, it is easy to lose sight of your goals and begin to aimlessly wander. It's hard enough to identify goals, but it can seem impossible to decide what belongs at the top of your list. There are so many distracting choices out there. Some call this "paralysis through analysis." To avoid this, stick to three or four goals at a time. Write them down, and check them off when you accomplish them. It will also help if you keep the four categories of goals in balance. These are short term, long term, serious, and fun goals.

The most important part of a goal is the *launch,* initiating the action required to move in the direction of the goal. Action is a source of great excitement and may be at times your only source of excitement. It shatters the "feel like nothing" syndrome.

Without goals, you are more apt to float on the whims and currents that randomly pass through your life. Compare it to river rafting. If you don't paddle the raft, it will spin around and bounce from rock to rock, shore to shore, and eventually get hung up somewhere or sink. However, if you exert a little effort and paddle, you gain control of the raft and avoid obstacles. Paddling gives the raft the power to move faster

than the current, which is the secret to changing direction quickly. Put some friends onboard,
paddle together, and now you have the power
of synergy and acceleration. You are on your
own "life raft." The paddle is in your hands, so
don't forget to use it.

Urgency and Motivation

There is old wisdom that says that you are born
with a number stamped on your forehead. This
is the number of days you get to live on this
planet. Do you have any idea what that number is or what number you are on today? If a
book were written on your life, how interesting
would it be to read? Is the first half filled with
adventure, insights, and accomplishments only
to have the story wear thin and plod to the pre-
dictable conclusion. Whoa! Your book of life is
like the glass of water that is half full. There's
more, lots more! The story should continue
growing and the glass should continue filling
with the abundance of the universe until the
last chapter is written. Your book of life will be
more interesting if you go out on a full glass
running over rather than on one that's run dry.

Taking Action

One of the definitions of insanity is *continuing to do what you have been doing in the same way and expecting a different result.* With this thought in mind, perhaps it's time to try something different. Don't fear change. Change is inevitable and an essential law of nature.

The following action strategies are based on taking a more proactive approach to your life in an effort to keep you healthier and more in balance. Add the following actions, especially aerobic breathing, to the MH breathing exercise and you will experience a powerful turnaround toward clarity. However, if you are in the throes of an MH and are experiencing impaired balance or other symptoms, approach these activities with caution or wait until the MH is over.

If MH stress continues to persist day after day, it is time to take evasive action. As soon as you are able, participate in some enjoyable diversions and spend more time in friendlier environments. Walk away from the gloom of idleness or stress. Contemplate this critical question: Just how big is "your world" right now? When your world becomes too small and routine, MH stress can easily overrun you. You can counteract this with the stimulation of travel. *Travel cleans the mind.* Don't get stuck, get moving, even if it's only a small day trip.

You can stimulate yourself through ideas, dreams, and goals, but beyond that you must find stimulation in the life around you, through your work, people, and nature. If you are feeling empty there is only one thing to do, get out there. *We are all conduits for life to flow through. It is this flow that stimulates us and makes us feel more alive.* Get out there and let the life force of the universe flow through you.

Breathing Aerobically

More than anything else your body needs oxygen. Oxygen plays a major role in healing infection and disease in the body. One of the bad habits I discovered about myself was that I repressed my breathing during and after stressful occurrences. My breath became so shallow that it momentarily stopped at times. My diaphragm muscles below the lungs tensed up drastically restricting inhalation. This created shallow breathing and a low oxygen environment in my body.

If your diaphragm and lung muscles feel sore when you take a really big breath, it's a sure sign that this area is too tight and needs to relax.

An activity or exercise that opens up the lungs and gets them pumping is a great way to counteract restricted breathing and tension. Exercise oxygenates the blood, whose primary function is to deliver that oxygen to the cells so they can fight disease and maintain health. I say forget the treadmill or the gym. Go outside, regardless of the weather. Stimulate your senses, excite your spirit, and rejuvenate your mind. *Nature cleans the spirit.* Pick up the pace and join in that wonderful child-like activity called "play." Breathe in oxygen and health, and breathe out stress. Movement will stimulate your cardiovascular system, bringing your mind and body together as one. Runners, cyclists, swimmers, and other athletes experience a sense of euphoria during and after aerobic exercise. In this super-oxygenated state, your brain is capable of phenomenal crystalline thought that produces ideas and solutions that were not there before. *Aerobic breathing cleans the emotions.*

For many people, the urge to exercise or stay active is not so much about getting in shape as about oxygenating themselves back into that "zone" where stress and stagnation melt away and are replaced with a sense of confidence and strength. Vigorous exercise will reinforce a general sense of harmony and well being in all aspects of your life. Exercise also burns up stress-generated hormones that might be circulating in the bloodstream and replaces them with "feel good" chemicals like endorphins.

Everyday, people around the world finish work and have an overwhelming sensation that they need to somehow "unwind." Many times, this sensation is really a craving by the body for more oxygen. After a stressful day of shallow or repressed breathing, your body's oxygen level will fall below normal and send an "add oxygen" signal to the brain. Learn to interpret this signal accurately and add the oxygen to your body through exercise to re-energize yourself.

Using Your Voice

Don't forget to use your voice. Stress and repressed breathing can start a negative chain reaction that begins with a verbal shutdown, which promotes the internalization and exaggeration of negative feelings, which in turn causes a stress-hormone release within your body, which then may lead to an MH attack. If you are more vocally *assertive* (not aggressive) with stressful events, you can break this negative chain reaction while clarifying and confirming the issues in your mind as well as in the minds of others. Repressed responses can bring you to a standstill, even though everything else around you continues to move forward. The voice is a wonderful thing; use it, don't lose it. Maintain your voice by joining a singing group, chanting, taking up yodeling, reading out loud to a child, joining an acting or voice class, cheering on your favorite team, or rendezvousing with boisterous friends who make you laugh. Whatever it might be, reassert your primal need to speak, sing, or roar.

Getting Adequate Sleep

Adequate sleep is the basis for good health. Sleep reduces stress, thereby helping you avoid MHs. Sleep rejuvenates the body, especially the brain and nervous system. After a day or two with little sleep, you will have difficulty concentrating on or performing routine tasks. Without sleep, you can easily be distracted. Feeling sleepy throughout the day is a sure sign that you need more sleep. Consuming caffeine to override this basic need is only a temporary fix. Some medical studies suggest that the body is geared to have a midday sleep period in addition to normal sleep at night. For centuries many cultures have included an afternoon nap in their daily routine. If you feel tired day after day, try a ten-minute "power nap" during the lunch hour. Also try to improve the quality of your sleep at night through daily exercise. My nightly routine includes some favorite stretches before bed. This helps me fall asleep quickly. Oversleeping in the morning to catch up is not effective for everyone because it may be very shallow sleep, which is not truly restful. If you feel you can't turn off your mind at night to fall asleep, try the MH breathing exercise to empty and relax the brain.

Drinking Enough Water

It amazes me that so many people live in a mild state of dehydration day after day. The body is about 60 percent water. It is essentially a steam engine that requires two liters of fresh water a day to function optimally. When your hydration level falls too low, your body fluids become more viscous (like honey), which stresses body functions and reduces your body's ability to optimally maintain itself. A stuffed up nose, bad breath, thick or dried saliva at the corners of your mouth, bright yellow urine, heavy underarm odor, and cracked skin next to fingernails are all indicators that you need more water. If toxins are not able to exit the body efficiently through the urine stream, they increase odor in the breath vapor and sweat. If you do not drink enough water, your mental, physical, and emotional performance levels will be compromised —whether you are the athlete or the spectator, the child or the adult.

Morning is the most important time to start drinking water because it immediately replaces fluids just eliminated by the body. Sooner or later, you will realize it is easier to periodically chug down twelve ounces of room temperature water rather than sipping it throughout the day. *Water cleans the body.* When you feel thirsty, don't ignore it. It's not time for just any beverage; it's time to hydrate first with water. Sodas, beer, coffee, and the like are only supplements to water. Water keeps the steam engine from overheating.

Applying MH Acupressure

Acupressure is a massage technique of applying intermittent pressure to tender areas of the body. For those who suffer from MHs, these areas include: the temples, eyebrows, and top of the head. These are locations where pain builds during the MH onset phase. Acupressure is an immediate and direct way to soothe the sore nerves around these areas. Once you massage around and find a sore spot, apply pressure with a fingertip or knuckle for ten seconds, pause, and then apply pressure again. You might also try using acupressure in the abdominal area just below the chest bones in order to relax the diaphragm and abdominal muscles. This may improve your breathing capacity. Five repetitions is enough to stimulate a sore spot, relaxing constricted muscles and swollen nerves, and renewing the flow of healing energy within your body. The body is repairing and healing itself twenty-four hours a day. Acupressure allows you to direct the healing flow to where it is needed.

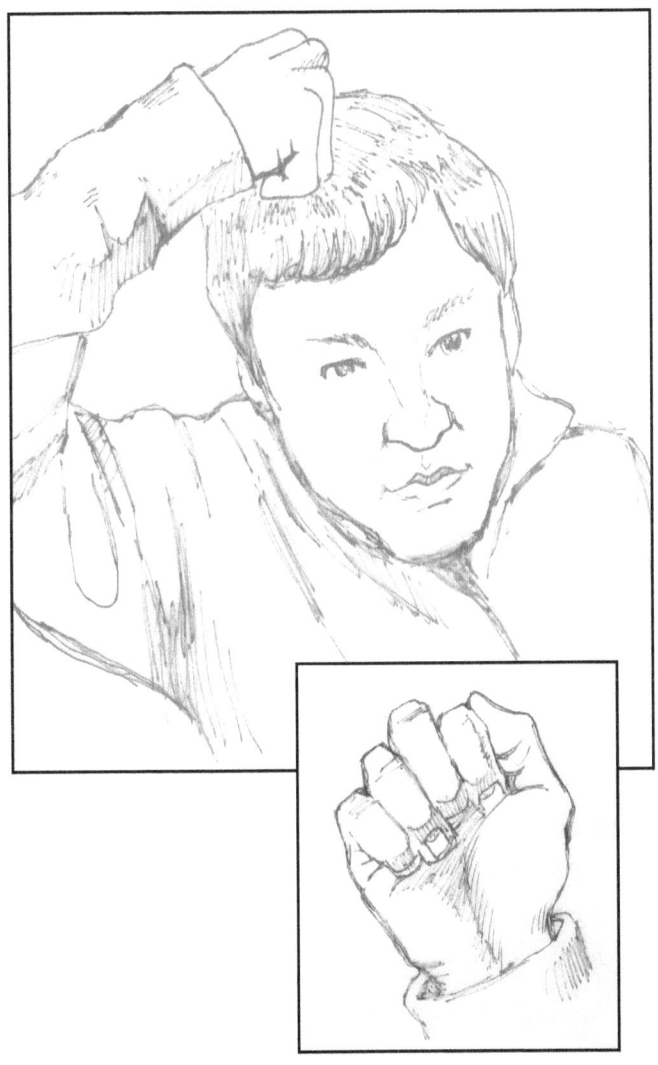

Laughing and Health

According to an old saying, "There are no guarantees in life." On the contrary, there *is* a guarantee: *Laughter is the secret to happiness.* You cannot be happy without laughing, and you cannot laugh without feeling happy! All kinds of good things happen when you laugh. Your body releases wonderful chemicals like endorphins that heal you and make you feel good. Laughter encourages other people to smile and laugh along with you. Laughter is an audible, physical, and emotional expression of happiness. It opens up the lungs with big happy breaths, illuminates facial expressions, uplifts the spirit, and makes your body resonate with positive vibrations. It is extremely contagious because everyone loves it and wants to do it, especially children. It has no age, cultural, or belief boundaries. *Laughter is one of the sterling common denominators of all human beings that can never be lost or outgrown.* A basic law of nature applies to laughing, it works best when it is shared with others. Cultivate friendships with those who make you laugh for they are most precious. You will be healthier, happier, and live longer with regular doses of laughter.

Staying Balanced

A healthy life is the result of "maintaining balance" one day to the next. You must choose to live life rather than to simply exist. Every day counts, every day is important. Life will knock you off balance sometimes, but the trick is to re-center yourself as quickly as possible. I have used three steps to regain a robust life free from the control of reoccurring MHs.

- First, when stress and tension build up and begin to disrupt my peace of mind and threaten me with an MH, I know I can rely on the MH breathing exercise to neutralize the MH at the onset and return to normal. It is an incredible tool for better health and a natural alternative to medication.

- Second, I use various coping strategies focused on making a continual decision to drop my negative reaction and *respond* positively to what comes my way. Adapting, embracing and being part of change keeps me moving forward. I practice self-encouragement by using and listening to my positive, reassuring voice, which brings immediate results through the law of attraction. Good thoughts cause good vibrations and attract good things. This creates a new outlook for me, one of insight, clarity, and optimism. When I have a positive perception of life, it greatly reduces what I perceive as stressful and accelerates the attainment of my goals.

■ Finally, I follow action strategies that create excitement and exhilaration in my weekly routines. I've learned to take the time to go outside and breathe big, live full, sleep deep, cheer, and laugh! It's okay to play and be creative. By getting out there and doing what I enjoy, I reinforce my sense of confidence, strength, and satisfaction.

One of my dad's favorite sayings was, "You have friends you haven't even met yet". So go find them. Share some laughter, activity, and quality time with them. Explore the wonders of nature and realize the benefit of maintaining a healthy oxygen-rich balance in your body. Remember, *the meaning of life is greater happiness. It's all about feeling more alive.* Life is not a battle. Life is not a race. Life … is the next breath you take.

Notes

Notes

Notes

Notes

Notes

Notes

About the Author

Allan McMullen has been studying the human body's innate ability to heal itself for most of his life. Originally from the mountains of northern New Mexico, he was an athlete and professional skier in his younger years and had his share of injuries. With the help of stitches, plaster and fiberglass casts, and mental focus, his body's healing process prevailed each time. Mentored and guided by a few key doctors and healers over the years, he has always heard the basic echoing premise that "the body is perfectly capable of healing itself; all we have to do is help it do its job." With this resolute belief, he turned his healing focus toward his migraine headache problem. As one of millions who suffered from this ailment with no known cure, it was a journey into the unknown.

However, with his breakthrough discovery of resistance breathing and his personal in-depth research, the journey was a successful one.

While working on this book, he considered many issues, especially the connectivity of the human inner voice with the outer world and how balance is synonymous with health. The goal was achieved: freedom from MHs. Once again, the premise that the human body can heal itself proved to be true.